THE
POCKET
DOCTOR

To your
good health

Mick O'Rourke
12/96

THE POCKET DOCTOR
500 Medical Tips You Need to Stay Healthy and Calm Your Fears

Michael A. LaCombe, M.D.

Andrews and McMeel
A Universal Press Syndicate Company
Kansas City

THE POCKET DOCTOR Copyright © 1996 by Michael LaCombe, M.D. All rights reserved. Printed in the United States of America. No part of this book may be used or reproduced in any manner whatsoever except in the case of reprints in the context of reviews. For information, write Andrews and McMeel, a Universal Press Syndicate Company, 4520 Main Street, Kansas City, Missouri 64111.

Library of Congress Cataloging-in-Publication Data

LaCombe, Michael.
    The pocket doctor : 500 medical tips you need to stay healthy and calm your fears / [Michael LaCombe].
      p.   cm.
    ISBN 0-8362-2166-4
    1. Medicine, Popular—Miscellanea.   I. Title.
RC82.L33 1996
610—dc20   96-7960
                                                            CIP

ATTENTION: SCHOOLS AND BUSINESSES

Andrews and McMeel books are available at quantity discounts with bulk purchase for educational, business, or sales promotional use. For information, please write to: Special Sales Department, Andrews and McMeel, 4520 Main Street, Kansas City, Missouri 64111.

For Margaret Mary

In my twenty years of medical practice I've answered all sorts of questions from patients: questions about the dark fear of cancer and questions in the hospital late at night about when death will come; questions hesitant and apologetic, about sex and marriage, life and death, youth and growing old; questions about innocent rashes and lethal moles, about innocuous bleeding and bleeding from deep inside; questions in the privacy of the examination room and questions never asked at all.

Here are some answers.

1. Your allotted time on earth is
   diminished neither by gardening
   nor by fly-fishing.

2. *What wound did ever heal but by*
   degrees?

   Othello

3. Cortisone can be a dangerous drug. Use it with care and under supervision. A colleague once said it is the only drug that will allow you to walk to your own funeral.

4. By age eighteen, 65 percent of males and 51 percent of females are sexually active.

5. Shots your adolescent should have before leaving the nest:
- mumps, measles, rubella booster
- tetanus booster
- hepatitis B series

6. If you forget something, then
   remember it later on, you do not
   have Alzheimer's. You're normal.
   Relax!

7. You cannot catch AIDS from
   saliva, nor from toilet seats, nor
   from mosquitoes.

8. Beware of medical entrepreneurs in shopping malls. They will offer to "sound" your arteries at no charge, let you listen to the "noise," warn you about the danger of stroke, and lead you down the path to unnecessary surgery.

9. Acute back pain only in the back and not traveling to the buttocks or legs is very common. You don't need a month off work. Prolonged bed rest is unnecessary. You do not need X rays. Take aspirin or Tylenol®, learn how to protect your back, and get some instruction in back exercises from your doctor's office.

10. There is no cure for the common cold. Antibiotics are of no value, and may actually make things worse. Drugs used to lessen the symptoms contain derivatives of cysteine, allinin, and capsaicin. That's why your Jewish mother's chicken soup can be so comforting (provided she throws in some garlic and a few chili peppers).

11. Preventive medicine for people over sixty-five:

- a medical history and a physical examination by your doctor, including a blood pressure check, a check on vision and hearing, a breast examination, and a pelvic and rectal examination
- mammograms

- a flu shot, a pneumonia shot, and an updated tetanus shot
- blood tests for cholesterol and sugar and a urine test
- an EKG
- a Pap smear
- a test for fecal blood with a sigmoidoscopy

A routine chest X ray is no longer necessary.

12. Thank your doctor.

13. An adequate medical history
and physical examination take
longer than twenty minutes,
managed care organizations
notwithstanding.

14. Your risk of HIV infection through heterosexual activity goes up dramatically if you have another sexually transmitted disease (gonorrhea, syphilis, chlamydia, genital herpes).

15. The hand tremor you get when you reach for something or attempt to balance that fifth cup of coffee is the result of stimulants, stress, or fatigue. It is not a sign of Parkinson's disease. Early Parkinson's tremor occurs at *rest*, not with activity.

16. Sooner or later, on some form or other, you will be asked if you have ever been treated for a psychiatric disease. Always answer "No." There are two reasons why:

- most so-called psychiatric disease is really a biochemical problem, and
- it is none of their damn business

17. Hair loss in women is almost always the result of stress, and is temporary. Rogaine® won't help. (It is of very little help in men, for that matter.)

18. Don't waste your money on power bars and power drinks boasting OKG, Vanadyl, Creatine, etc. For rehydration after exercise, drink water.

19. Get a Pap smear every year until you are sixty-five. Then, every three years.

20. Major depression is more common than you think. Learn the signs: lack of interest, hypersomnia (excessive sleeping), weight loss or gain, loss of energy, inability to concentrate, preoccupation with death.

21. Urinary incontinence can be treated with medication and exercise. Remember, try that before you submit to unnecessary surgery.

22. Antioxidant vitamins slow down retinal degeneration and the progression of Parkinson's disease. See tip no. 380.

23. Hypochondriasis can be a symptom
of depression, neurosis, or
domestic violence.

24. Wear polarized sunglasses to help
prevent cataracts.

25. Yes, you should consider hormone replacement at menopause. By all means talk to your doctor about this.

26. Sudden vertigo (feelings of spinning, room moving, imbalance) is common, frightening, and most often caused by a virus. It is very rarely a symptom of impending stroke.

27. It is not unusual for college coeds to gain thirty pounds during the freshman year.

28. You cannot lose weight, and keep it off, without exercising.

29. Pink-eye is very common, very contagious, and very easily treated. Symptoms: your eyes get red and itchy. There is drainage, and the lids are crusted together in the morning.

30. Glaucoma is very rare before age forty.

31. Get a flu shot if you are over sixty-five, chronically ill, or cannot possibly afford to miss work. Don't get one if you are allergic to eggs.

32. Sinusitis is not just a runny nose. Pain over the sinuses (the cheek-bones or forehead) with congestion and foul nasal discharge, often with fever, means bacterial infection of the sinuses. For this, you need antibiotics.

33. If you are hoarse for longer than two weeks, you need to see an ear, nose, and throat specialist. If you are a smoker, get there fast.

34. A runny nose can be caused by allergy, medications (including birth-control pills), heat, cold, cooking odors, perfume, stress, sexual excitement, and polyps induced by aspirin, as well as by the common cold.

35. Premature ejaculation is very
common in young men. Stop
worrying! Your partner can easily
help you control it. Learn how
from your doctor.

36. Asthma is common. Its only
symptom may be a chronic
recurring cough. Asthma is easily
diagnosed, easily treated.

37. Lifelong smokers can lose up to
fifteen years of life expectancy.

38. Secondhand smoking (passive smoking) is potentially dangerous. Spouses of smokers have one-and-a-half to two times the risk of lung cancer, and children of smokers have an increased risk of asthma, respiratory infection, and ear infections.

39. See your doctor for influenza if you have a chronic illness, or if you get increasing fever, productive cough, shortness of breath, and chest pain.

40. Show a good nurse your appreciation.

41. Hypertension is not "hyper-tension."
High blood pressure does not
always give you feelings of stress
or tension. Most hypertension has
no symptoms whatsoever. Which is
why it is called the silent killer.

42. Call the nurses' station at your hospital. Ask which patient never has visitors, never gets mail. Send him or her a card or flowers or, best of all, pay a visit.

43. When is acute chest pain not heart pain (angina)? It takes a savvy doctor to tell the difference. It's never "just gas" until your doctor says so.

44. Sex after a heart attack? Here's the story: Make sure you have a stress exercise test before leaving the hospital. If you can get your heart rate to 120 beats per minute without problems, you can safely resume sexual activity *with your spouse or usual partner.*

45. If you have a heart murmur, take antibiotics before dental work or surgery.

46. A leg cramp when walking that stops when you rest is a sign of poor arterial circulation. Common in smokers. See a doctor.

47. Calf pain and swelling may
    indicate phlebitis (a blood clot in
    the vein). You need to be seen.
    Today.

48. Most pain or difficulty on
    swallowing is not cancer. Cancer of
    the esophagus is rare.

49. Treat dyspepsia with dietary changes (avoid caffeine, alcohol, tobacco, fatty foods). Then try antacids for a week or so. Then see your doctor.

50. Diarrhea alternating with constipation, cramping abdominal pain, fatigue, and nausea all constitute the irritable bowel syndrome. It is very, very common; perhaps as many as 20 percent of us have it. Before seeing a gastroenterologist, try bran cereal once a day, avoid caffeine and carbonated beverages, and begin an aerobic exercise program.

51. Treat hemorrhoids with hot baths, stool softeners (mineral oil, Haley's MO®), and increased dietary fiber. You don't need Preparation H . . . and don't read on the toilet.

52. Gallstones are common. A quarter of women over fifty have them. If they are not causing symptoms, leave them there. Unless you have diabetes or are a Native American woman, in which case, get a few opinions.

53. The best, least risky permanent contraception for a woman is still vasectomy for her partner.

54. Impotence after vasectomy is very
uncommon, is always
psychological, and is always
treatable.

55. Vasectomy does not change
testosterone levels.

56. Increased frequency of urination with pain on passing urine, with or without bloody urine, and without back pain or significant fever is *cystitis*, or a bladder infection. It can be treated over the phone, without a urine test, with a prescription for antibiotics.

57. A kidney stone can be the worst pain there is. Excruciating pain in the flank, traveling around to the lower abdomen on that side, and then to the groin, occasionally with bloody urine, should drive the victim to the emergency room. Don't try to tough it out.

58. The arthritis of advancing age, *osteoarthritis*, occurs in 90 percent of people over fifty. It is from the wear-and-tear of the "gristle" of the joints, and is never crippling.

59. Ice or hot packs? Ice for the first twenty-four hours, then heat. For sprains, bursitis, tendonitis, or pulled muscles.

60. Antibiotics, birth-control pills, obesity, nylon underwear, diabetes—these predispose you to vaginal yeast infection. Symptoms are: itching, pain on intercourse, and a cottage cheese–like discharge. For a first infection with these symptoms, treat it yourself with Monistat® or Gyn-lotrimin®

vaginal cream at bedtime for three
to seven days. Sexual partners
without symptoms do not need to
be treated.

61. If you are over thirty-five and
smoke, don't use birth-control
pills.

62. There is absolutely no scientific evidence to support the connection between silicon breast implants and disease. In fact, there is compelling evidence to the contrary.

63. Abnormal uterine bleeding in girls
ages eleven to sixteen is from
failure to ovulate. Very common in
adolescence, it is nothing to worry
about.

64. PMS is a physiologic disorder, not
a psychological aberration.
Effective therapy exists. Talk to
your doctor.

65. *In general, mankind, since the improvement of cookery, eats twice as much as nature requires.*

Benjamin Franklin

66. The bigger the ad, the better the drug? No. Aspirin is still the best, most miraculous drug ever discovered.

67. Transient, fleeting blindness in one eye *must* be investigated by a physician. Let me repeat: Reassurance over the phone about this symptom will not save your vision or prevent a serious stroke. You must see a physician.

68. If you have a sore throat, fever, swollen neck glands, pus on the tonsils, and no cough, the chances are about fifty-fifty you have a strep throat and require antibiotics.

69. Leg cramps at night are extremely common, and almost never associated with disease. Try vitamin E (see tip no. 380), quinine 300 mg. tablet (over-the-counter, fifteen cents a pill), and calf muscle stretching exercises. You shouldn't need a doctor for this one.

70. Unless it's bloody, any nipple discharge is *rarely* due to cancer.

71. Thyroid problems are common, especially in women, and especially after fifty.

72. Many elderly people who live alone are malnourished. These "tea-and-toasters" are victims of depression, waning appetite, social isolation, and poverty.

73. Fear of crowds, panic about big parties, the tendency toward becoming a shut-in—these are kinds of panic disorders for which excellent medical treatment now exists. Xanax®, for example, can work miracles.

74. It is not critical that you know your blood type. Better that you know your cholesterol.

75. When you donate blood—as you should—you will be checked for anemia, for HIV infection, and for hepatitis.

76. Anxiety or "nerves" is extremely
common. It should be treated with
medication—there is no reason to
suffer. Resulting dependence on
the drugs used to treat it is very
uncommon—only 1 percent of
patients so treated become
dependent.

77. The best drugs for treatment of anxieties are the benzodiazepines: Xanax®, Serax®, Valium®, Ativan®, Librium®, Tranxene®, Klonopin®. Don't believe what the media tells you about these medications. Believe your doctor.

78. When you read about the presumed horrors of a popular drug—Valium® or Prozac®, for example—remember that corporate America is in fierce competition.

79. Have your own doctor. Ensure that you do so while you are well; when you are ill, your doctor will be there for you.

80. Reflux of acid into the esophagus at night can be the cause of chronic cough, hoarseness, or asthma.

81. Battering is the leading cause of
injury to women ages fifteen to
forty-four years. Sixty-eight
percent of victims want to tell their
doctors. Only four percent of
doctors ask.

82. Can't sleep? Cut out the naps, exercise earlier in the day, no caffeine or nicotine after mid-afternoon, don't read in bed. Call back if no success and we'll try a short course of sleeping pills.

83. Grief and bereavement are *normal.*
And the symptoms—anxiety,
depression, insomnia, loss of
appetite—should be treated. *Of
course* you should call for help with
this!

84. The CAGE test for alcoholism:

- ever felt the need to *C*ut down?
- ever been *A*nnoyed by criticism of your drinking?
- ever felt *G*uilty about your drinking?
- ever had a morning *E*ye-opener?

Two or more yesses equal an 80 to 100 percent probability of alcoholism.

85. Shingles is common. Half of us get it by age eighty-five. Caused by the chicken pox virus, it produces burning pain in one area of the body on one side only, with a rash and clusters of tiny blisters that crust over. Shingles on the face must be examined by a physician. Those not previously infected with chicken pox can catch it from people with active shingles.

86. Hives from stress, heat, cold, and exercise are especially common in redheads.

87. Stung by a bee? Stung before, but this time your entire arm is swollen? Better come in to the office.

88. What patients want most from doctors is conversation. Don't expect to get it in a managed care organization with obligatory ten-minute appointments.

89. Young athletes who die suddenly during competition have a family history of such events and a prior history of fainting during exercise. After a good screening physical, let your son or daughter play ball.

90. If you are over fifty, take one aspirin every other day.

91. The best person to ask about drug interactions is your pharmacist.

92. Did you get an adequate breast examination by your doctor? It takes at least two minutes to examine a single breast adequately.

93. The American Cancer Society recommends annual PSA testing (for prostate cancer) for all men age fifty and over.

94. Any elderly person who faints should be evaluated by a physician.

95. Edema (swelling of the legs) is very common. Causes: varicose veins, medications, heat, heart and lung disease, liver and kidney disease.

96. Don't climb Mt. Washington in July without a pack full of winter clothing and emergency rations.

97. Don't treat frostbite with ice, alcohol, or nicotine. Warm gently.

98. Puncture wounds from human bites are potentially dangerous and need treatment with antibiotics.

99. You're never too old to exercise.

100. There *is* effective drug therapy for obesity. Refer your doctor to Weintraub's research in *Clinical Pharmacologic Therapy,* 1992; 51:581–5.

101. In some areas of the United States, 50 percent of prostitutes carry HIV infection.

102. Middle-aged people who quit smoking gain three years in life expectancy.

103. Bring all of your pill bottles with you to your doctor's appointment. Always. Even those bottles from that other doctor . . .

104. Leg cramps at night are not a circulatory problem. Not serious. Don't worry. See tip no. 69.

105. Would that women worried as much about breast cancer as they do about cholesterol.

106. Sudden, sharp pain in the chest that catches you, limits your breathing, and is made worse by deep breathing is a blood clot to the lungs until your doctor tells you otherwise.

107. *Middle age has been said to be the time of a man's life when, if he has two choices for an evening, he takes the one that gets him home earlier.*

Alvan L. Barach

108. Fever, sore throat, and markedly swollen glands in someone age fifteen to twenty-five is most likely infectious mononucleosis, *not* AIDS.

109. Compulsive handwashing and other obsessions (repeatedly checking the stove, the fire, etc.) are now eminently treatable with prescription medication. One drug, Anafranil®, can work miracles with this disorder, sometimes abolishing it overnight.

110. *It is the mind . . . not the limbs, that taints by long sitting.*

Charles Lamb

111. Headaches that recur over time, with intervals of pain-free periods, are not due to brain tumors.

112. What signals do victims of
domestic violence give to friends
and neighbors?

- increasing social isolation
- inappropriate clothing to hide
  bruises
- substance abuse

113. Small, blind pouches in the colon (diverticulosis) are very common in middle age and old age. Prevention and treatment both include a high-fiber diet. Bran cereal is best. It needn't taste good to be effective. All-Bran® and Bran-Buds® are cheapest, have the least fat and sugar, and will do just fine.

114. If you do have bona fide *rheumatoid arthritis* and your doctor first recommends aspirin, be reassured you have a good doctor.

115. If, after drinking from a pristine
mountain stream, you develop
explosive, watery diarrhea, you
have "beaver fever" or giardiasis.
Quinacrine clears it up quickly.

116. Doctors don't like patients with lists. Bring yours along anyway, and apologize for it. Put what is bothering you most at the top of the list; don't bring it up only when your doctor is leaving the room.

117. Asthma is common, is underdiagnosed, and is easily treated. You can "get it" at any age. No history of allergy necessary.

118. A heart attack characteristically involves intense, overwhelming chest pain described as a heavy weight or pressure, often with sweating, nausea, shortness of breath, and fear. The pain may travel to the arms, wrists, jaw, back, or shoulder. Pain of this sort is a true emergency!

119. Get stitches if you can't close the mouth of the wound with a couple of Steri-strips®—and especially if the cut is on the face.

120. Any cut across the border of the lip (the vermilion border) requires sutures to prevent an ugly scar.

121. Get a tetanus booster every ten years or at the time of injury, whichever comes first.

122. Learn the Heimlich maneuver.

123. Common contact allergens that can produce a rash: suntan lotions, glue, cosmetics, latex, perfumes, toothpaste, nickel, leather, plastics, neoprene, wool, hair dye, shampoos, topical medications, rubber, topical antibiotics.

124. A fever of 105°F without sweating can mean heatstroke. Move the person out of the sun to a cool, preferably air-conditioned place and call the rescue squad.

125. The cardinal symptoms of carbon monoxide poisoning are headache and confusion. If you wake up with a headache and find a family member hard to arouse, get everyone out of the house immediately.

126. Forgetting to take your
medication, wondering whether to
double up on it, not knowing how
to compensate for the lapse—
legitimate reasons to call your
doctor's office.

127. A common mistake of diabetics on insulin: not feeling well, so not eating well, so better cut back on the insulin dose. Such reasoning often leads to diabetic coma.

128. When taking a rectal temperature, *never* let go of the thermometer.

129. Penicillin-allergic people may cross-react with a host of other medications. Likewise, aspirin-allergic people.

130. Much alternative medicine has great merit. But not yeast allergy theories and rotation diets.

131. Treatment of gout does not necessarily mean daily medication.

132. Teen girls who hold "ear-lobe piercing" parties are at increased risk of hepatitis.

133. Chest pain that occurs at rest, varies with position and posture, and tends to diminish with activity is not heart pain.

134. Scalp wounds always bleed profusely. Stay calm. Gentle pressure with a clean towel is all that is required until you get to the emergency room.

135. It is very, very uncommon to become "crippled up" with arthritis, and even then, corrective surgery works miracles.

136. For a painful shoulder, begin
treatment with aspirin (or one of
its alternatives—see tip no. 450)
and continue a gentle range of
motion exercises in the shower or
hot tub to avoid a frozen shoulder.

137. The best prevention for osteoporosis is weight-bearing exercise. A lifelong habit of daily walking will do it.

138. Never attempt to remove a foreign body embedded in the eyeball. Cover the eye with a sterile pad and get the person to the emergency room.

139. All things in moderation. It won't kill you to have that end-cut of prime rib every few months.

140. In adults, a fever of 101°F or more lasting three days or more demands medical attention. A fever together with confusion and a stiff neck is a medical emergency (meningitis).

141. A good slap on the back treats *no* medical emergency; use the Heimlich maneuver.

142. Never give aspirin to children with a fever. Use Tylenol®.

143. The pain from blunt trauma to the
scrotum lasts about an hour, and is
severe. If it persists longer than
that and/or there is significant
swelling, seek emergency help.
Any penetrating wound to the
scrotum is an emergency.

144. Scabies is common, for all groups of people and in all age groups. You get it through shared clothing or infested bed sheets, not by being dirty and poor. Severe itching at night, ultimately afflicting the entire family, is the cardinal symptom. Wash clothing and bedsheets in hot water, and use Kwell® as directed.

145. You can donate blood five times a
year without any ill effects.

146. If you have chronic bad breath, see
your dentist.

147. Get over-the-counter ointments for canker sores.

148. You do not need iodine pills to prevent goiter.

149. Combining medications in one single pill is a bad idea. It's more expensive, and makes it impossible to adjust dosages.

150. Depression, lethargy, dry skin, brittle hair, and weight gain are early symptoms of an underactive thyroid gland.

151. Heart disease is underdiagnosed in women.

152. Beware of laxatives.

153. Keep a volume of poetry at the bedside.

154. Learn to appreciate classical music.

155. To increase your endurance, increase the length of your workout rather than its intensity.

156. *Allow patients to escape with the slightest attack of surgery your skill can supply.*

Robert Tuttle Morris

157. A woman with troublesome fatigue may be iron-deficient without having an anemia.

158. Fullness and pain in the ear, fever,
and decreased hearing indicate a
middle ear infection. Antibiotic
pills, not drops, are the answer.

159. No adolescent need be permanently scarred by acne. One cure that doesn't require a prescription: use a drying soap (Fostex® or Pernox®) in the morning and 10 percent benzoyl peroxide at bedtime. Avoid lotions, creams, and makeup on the face. This approach is highly successful, but if not, see your doctor. There is no connection between acne and foods (chocolate, fatty foods, etc.).

160. Brand-name aspirin and generic aspirin differ only in cost.

161. Some truth in advertising: "Low cholesterol" does not make it healthy. Heroin is low in cholesterol.

162. When making hotel reservations, ask first about their fitness center.

163. The hard lumps in the palm of the hand are called Dupuytren's contractures. They can cause a flexion deformity of a finger and can easily be removed surgically.

164. These doctors do *not* have M.D. degrees: podiatrists, chiropractors, optometrists, osteopaths, clinical psychologists, veterinarians, nuclear physicists, dentists, and many oral surgeons.

165. After age forty, see an optometrist
every two years as a routine.

166. Early Hodgkin's disease is curable.

167. The cardinal symptoms of an over-active thyroid gland are: weight loss, sweating, jitteriness, diarrhea, tremor, increased appetite, palpitations, and intolerance to heat.

168. Varicose veins are best treated
with daily walking.

169. Painful external hemorrhoids can
best be treated with hot baths
twice a day.

170. Loss of the outside third of the eyebrows is caused by only two diseases: leprosy and underactive thyroid.

171. Uncontrollable leg jerking and twitching, especially at night, is called the restless legs syndrome; it is common, not serious, and treatable.

172. Drink six eight-ounce glasses of water a day. Coffee, tea, and juice don't count.

173. Severe pain in the heel—common in walkers and runners—is usually not a bone spur, but is called plantar fasciitis. Treat with a hard sole insert, and good arch support during the waking hours. Avoid surgery and injections!

174. It takes the average American couple thirty-eight minutes to reach orgasm. Slow down!

175. The average American couple has intercourse twice a week, but would prefer it more often. Yes, the woman too.

176. As you exercise and your muscles become stronger, stretching before exercise becomes extremely important.

177. The hot flashes of menopause will respond to hormone replacement. And you will lessen your risks of osteoporosis and coronary artery disease.

178. Learn the universal sign for choking: the hand clutched to the throat with the thumb and fingers extended.

179. Use of birth-control pills reduces lifetime risk of ovarian cancer by at least 25 percent.

180. Airplane cabins are pressurized to 9,000 feet. If you have emphysema, check with your doctor before flying.

181. Half of all people over fifty have a
hiatal hernia. It is almost always
not a problem unless heartburn
and chronic reflux lead to scarring
and a stricture.

182. Never use the threat of a
malpractice suit when negotiating
with a doctor.

183. If you have a suspicious mole that bears watching, have your doctor photograph it.

184. Those soft, brown, raised moles with a waxy surface found in advancing age are not pre-cancerous.

185. Have moles with more than two colors, or containing white or black, checked by a physician.

186. Antibiotics will not kill viruses.

187. Skin cancers from sun exposure
first start with a small, pale spot
having a brittle surface. A topical
cream, Efudex®, will clear up the
matter.

188. Antiviral drugs—acyclovir, Zovirax®, and others—will kill only a small number of viruses under certain limited conditions.

189. Always use the stairs when going up one or two flights.

190. Obese people with chronic fatigue, hypersomnia, and headaches, and who snore regularly, may have sleep apnea syndrome.

191. A doctor who feels the front of your neck from behind is looking for thyroid cancer. Good for her!

192. The price of an antibiotic is no measure of its worth.

193. The number of laboratory tests ordered is inversely proportional to the length of the visit with the doctor.

194. Always fasten your seatbelt.

195. Asymmetry of breasts, one slightly larger than the other, is extremely common in women.

196. In motorcycle accidents, helmeted riders go to the orthopedists. Those without, to the neurosurgeons or the morgue.

197. Ninety percent of all lung cancer is associated with cigarette smoking.

198. To remove an insect from the ear canal: Lay the person good ear down; pull the ear lobe up and back to straighten the ear canal; drop warm mineral oil into the ear to drown the insect and float it out.

199. Take a course in first aid.

200. Learn CPR.

201. Parkinson's disease under the age of fifty is extremely uncommon. Unless you are taking a medication that can produce the symptoms as a side effect, in which case it will go away when the medication is stopped. Or unless you use designer street drugs (MPTP), in which case it won't.

202. Surgery for peptic ulcers is
unheard-of today.

203. Asymptomatic genital herpes can
recur after years of a quiescent
phase. The presence of a genital
herpes ulcer does not have to
mean your spouse has been
cheating on you.

204. Tension headaches (that constant, unrelenting aching or pulling sensation in the neck, the back of the head, or the top of the skull) can last for weeks, produce feelings of light-headedness, and make concentrating difficult. They can be relieved by hot showers, exercise, distraction, and alcohol. Migraine headache cannot be so relieved.

205. Don't harangue your doctor for antibiotics to treat viral illnesses like colds and the flu.

206. Blood in the urine is always serious until your doctor says otherwise.

207. You cannot spot reduce. It is physiologically impossible. But if you commit to aerobic exercise, whether swimming or running or cycling or walking, you will lose the spare tire, the beer gut, and the cellulite.

208. Runners: Treat chronic knee pain with aspirin before and after exercise, and reduce your mileage until you recover.

209. Painful periods and painful breasts during menses are not psychological. Both respond well to ibuprofen (Motrin®, Advil®, Nuprin®), 400–600 mg. four times a day, rather than aspirin. Begin the pills at the start of menses.

210. Don't break the blister of a second-degree burn.

211. Your risk of heart attack returns to normal within five years of quitting smoking.

212. Two percent milk does *not* contain 2 percent of the fat of whole milk, but rather 62 percent. Any time you see "2 percent milk" hyped, think "62 percent."

213. Skim milk is the only true low-fat milk.

214. Most of the time the cause of hives is never found.

215. Hives caused by abrupt changes in body temperature—heat urticaria or cold urticaria—are fairly common, not serious, and usually easy to control.

216. In societies where diet is high in fiber and in vitamins A, C, E, D, and calcium, and low in fat and cholesterol, and where there is abstinence from alcohol and tobacco, colon cancer is very uncommon.

217. Alcoholism is a genetic disease devoid of any implicit moral presumption.

218. Anabolic (androgenic) steroids used by body builders can cause rapid liver failure and death.

219. Use allergy shots for seasonal hay
fever only as a last resort. Better
to avoid the offending ragweed or
use antihistamines and nasal
sprays for a limited period of time.

220. There are over two hundred viruses that can cause colds. You have to get immune to each one of them. Three or four colds per year is average.

221. Contrary to popular belief, X rays, CAT scanners, and MRIs reveal far less than does talking to the patient.

222. Charm, fluency, and bedside manner are no measure of medical expertise.

223. Losing weight is the toughest challenge one can face. It is more difficult than achieving abstinence from alcohol or tobacco, and much harder than daily exercise.

224. Dress to please others. Eat to please yourself.

225. Bad-tasting diet foods do not contain negative calories.

226. The world's great unsung hero is the inventor of the chocolate chip cookie.

227. Moderation in all things.

228. Alcoholics cannot engage in "controlled" drinking.

229. After years of practice and legions of patients, I have learned that the best treatment for alcoholism is Alcoholics Anonymous.

230. Pharmacists can "blister-pack" medications for patients who have trouble sticking to a schedule.

231. When you find a personal physician, you do not surrender responsibility for your own body.

232. With infertility, a third of the time it is the woman's problem, a third the husband's, and a third the couple's. Always start with a sperm count.

233. A patient can live with almost anything when supported by a loving family.

234. You cannot "catch" cancer. Touch
and hold your loved ones.

235. Almost every disease is explained
in a free brochure, available
through your doctor's office.

236. *The sooner patients can be removed from the depressing influence of general hospital life the more rapid their convalescence.*

Charles H. Mayo

237. If you have a runner's injury, see a doctor who runs.

238. Doctors are human. Just as with you, their sense of caring may be eclipsed by worry, fatigue, and the stress of the day.

239. Learn the difference between joy and pleasure.

240. Learn the difference between what is good and what is socially acceptable.

241. A blood pressure check is not a complete medical examination.

242. If you have heart disease, a supervised exercise program will reduce your risk of fatal heart attack by 20 percent

243. *The normal's the one thing you practically never get. That's why it's called the normal.*

W. Somerset Maugham

244. The most common cause of stroke in young people is recreational drug use —and not just the use of cocaine, but amphetamines and over-the-counter diet pills as well. Be careful!

245. In the elderly, disorders and disease caused by doctors and their medications (iatrogenesis) can occur as much as 40 percent of the time. If Grandma starts acting weirdly, have her medications checked.

246. Numbness and/or pain in the thumb and first two fingers is from a pinched nerve in the wrist (*Carpal tunnel syndrome*). Avoid the repetitive activity that may be causing it, use aspirin to reduce wrist swelling, and wear a light wrist splint until symptoms disappear. If they persist, it's time to see your doctor.

247. Diabetics: Have a podiatrist teach you good foot care.

248. Serious allergy to stinging insects can be treated effectively with allergy shots (immunotherapy).

249. If dark brown birthmarks run in
your family and you have inherited
the condition, get examined by a
dermatologist once a year.

250. There is no convincing evidence
that EBV infection (Epstein-Barr
virus, or mono virus) is linked to
the chronic fatigue syndrome.

251. Science has told us this: Three twenty-minute exercise sessions per week are far better for you than one hour on Saturday.

252. Buy a new toothbrush every three months.

253. Make time for exercise, and for family, and for reading, and yours will be a long, healthy, happy life.

254. Strong black coffee will not sober up a drunk, improve his awareness, or permit him to drive more safely. Take his car keys.

255. The good doctor helps a patient
sort out the difference between
wants and needs.

256. I have a patient/friend who
schedules his fly-fishing between
his thrice-weekly visits to the
kidney dialysis center. No self-pity
there!

257. After fifty, one worries less about psychological and more about physical problems. That shift of attention does not mean you are falling apart or getting ready to die.

258. Eat broccoli often.

259. Eat processed meats rarely.

260. Never eat red hot dogs, unless you're Grammy Feeney.

261. You can simplify the pain of indecision by always ordering fish when dining out.

262. Total joint replacement (hips, knees) is chiefly for the elderly. It is miraculous surgery.

263. The red, itchy rash in the groin—
common with athletes who hang
workout clothes in a locker rather
than wash them—can be cleared
up with Tinactin® or Lotrimin®.

264. Underarm rashes are usually from allergies—to deodorants or detergents and fabric softeners in clothing.

265. Cotton swabs do not belong in the ear canal.

266. Bake cookies, chocolate cake, and
pecan pie. It will educate you
about ingredients.

267. Air conditioners and dehumidifiers
can be a source of lung infection
and lung allergies.

268. The painless, bony lumps on the outermost finger joints of the elderly are harmless and not related to crippling arthritis.

269. You can facilitate your next doctor's visit by listing beforehand your present and past medications, allergies, prior hospitalizations and surgeries, and family history of disease.

270. If you are spared a rectal and
genital examination at your annual
physical examination, don't feel
relieved. Feel cheated.

271. Take your medicine.

272. Do not take aspirin with Coumadin®.

273. Do not take erythromycin with Seldane®.

274. Symptoms of the common cold develop gradually; of influenza, suddenly.

275. If your job entails standing for hours at a time, use a small foot rest to flex your hips alternatively. Saves your back.

276. No good doctor will ever be threatened by your desire for a second opinion.

277. Biking without a helmet is like in-line skating in Manhattan.

278. Think of your brain as a muscle. It needs daily exercise.

279. Television does not exercise the brain.

280. The safest way to lower cholesterol is through diet and exercise, not with medication.

281. Learn how to check for testicular cancer.

282. The common large lumpy veins in the left scrotum are harmless.

283. A brisk fifteen-minute walk each day equals 365 miles a year.

284. Two successive heavy irregular menses require a call to your doctor's office.

285. An increase in the frequency of nighttime urination can be an early sign of high blood pressure.

286. Cranberry juice does not treat a bladder infection.

287. For teenagers, delay in onset of
menstruation may be caused by too
much dieting or excessive
exercising.

288. The cardinal signs of anorexia nervosa are:

- depression
- loss of appetite
- inappropriate concerns over obesity
- weight loss in an extremely active teenager
- loss of a quarter of one's body weight without apparent illness

289. To treat athlete's foot, wash your
feet every day, dry thoroughly, dust
your feet with an over-the-counter
antifungal powder, put on *clean*
cotton socks, and wear shoes
dusted with the same powder.

290. Inflammation of the head of the penis may be the first sign of diabetes.

291. Unexplained painless bleeding in the urine is an early symptom of a bladder tumor.

292. In the elderly, shaking chills, high temperature, rapid pulse, and confusion and disorientation constitute a medical emergency. Most often pneumonia or urinary tract infection is the cause.

293. When a boil persists beyond three days, or when it causes a fever, it should be drained.

294. How to diagnose hip fracture in an elderly person: inability to bear weight; the leg will appear shortened; there will be an outward turning of the foot on the side of the fracture.

295. With acute bronchitis, here's when
to call your doctor:
- fever over 101°F
- chest pain on breathing
- shortness of breath at rest
- cough productive of thick,
  discolored sputum

296. Don't even think of having that bunion operated on unless it interferes with your day-to-day activity.

297. The food is always preferable to the vitamin. Nutrition encompasses far more than a jar of pills.

298. Never ignore black or bloody bowel movements. (But remember, iron and bismuth—Pepto-bismol®— cause black stools.)

299. Vaginal bleeding after menopause *always* requires a physician's examination.

300. The best first-line treatment for asthma is the handheld inhaler. Never pills.

301. Hyperventilation is usually brought on by anxiety or a panic attack. Sometimes spasm of the fingers happens as well. Have the person breathe into a paper bag while reassuring and calming the person. This is not an emergency.

302. Anytime you experience sudden, severe pain anywhere without any apparent cause—pain you have not experienced before—consult your doctor.

303. Pica—the craving for and eating of unusual substances—can indicate iron-deficiency anemia. Common picas: starch, sugar, clay, crushed ice, paper.

304. Toxic shock syndrome: sudden fever, vomiting, weakness, confusion, fainting, and a sunburnlike rash. Remove the tampon and get to the emergency room.

305. Avoid asbestos like the plague.

306. Avoid insecticides like the plague.

307. Avoid cigarettes like the plague.

308. Avoid sunburn. Use a sunblock
with a rating of at least SPF-15.

309. If you are young and otherwise healthy and you awake to find a small blood clot on a portion of the white of your eye, don't worry. This is common, will not progress, will not cover the iris or pupil, will not lead to blindness, and will take many days to disappear. If however, you have high blood pressure, get it checked within the next several days.

310. If your house is on a granite ledge, have your water and air checked for radon.

311. If you will be traveling to an area where "turista" abounds, get antibiotics and instructions from your doctor before you go.

312. Life is what is happening to you
while you are getting ready for
something else.

313. Diabetics should be screened at
least once a year for microscopic
amounts of protein in the urine. If
positive for this, you should be
treated with a specific blood
pressure pill called an ACE
inhibitor, even if you do not have
high blood pressure.

314. Get a home blood pressure monitor and learn how to use it.

315. Floss.

316. A change in climate will not provide a lasting cure for arthritis.

317. For-profit managed care organizations return as much as 40 percent profit to investors. Is that health care reform?

318. The logic of government: tobacco subsidies, yes; screening mammography, no.

319. Asking your doctor for a written excuse to obtain airline ticket refunds is asking your doctor to lie for you.

320. Birth-control pills do not increase your risk of breast cancer.

321. *The young man knows the rules, but the old man knows the exceptions. . . . The young man feels uneasy if he is not continually doing something to stir up his patient's internal arrangements. The old man takes things more quietly, and is much more willing to let well enough alone.*

Oliver Wendell Holmes

322. Women who smoke are at increased risk for early menopause.

323. Mitral valve prolapse, a benign heart murmur condition, is very common—perhaps as many as one in five young women have it. It can produce palpitations and chest pain for which medicine is very effective.

324. Infectious mononucleosis starts
with a fever and a severe sore
throat. Then comes the
overwhelming fatigue and
markedly swollen glands.

325. For motion sickness during travel,
get a prescription for scopolamine
patches. Very effective.

326. There is a blood test available to detect whether a woman carries the abnormal gene for muscular dystrophy.

327. Viruses can infect the heart. Runners who continue to train hard despite a viral illness are especially prone. You do not want this.

328. *It is part of the cure to wish to be cured.*

Seneca

329. True narcolepsy—uncontrollable spells of falling asleep at any time or place—is extremely rare. In twenty years I saw one patient with the disease.

330. Chronic nasal stuffiness can be
due to polyps, and they can be
caused by a sensitivity to aspirin.
Try avoiding aspirin as a first step.

331. To minimize jet lag, avoid caffeine and alcohol on the flight, and take a mild sleeping pill as soon as you board the plane to help you sleep during the flight.

332. Any head trauma resulting in an altered level of consciousness requires emergency medical attention.

333. At present (1995), the risk of HIV infection through blood transfusion is one in 225,000. But the risk of hepatitis can be as high as one in 3,000.

334. The secret to weight loss is aerobic exercise.

335. The cause of chronic fatigue syndrome is not known. Patients fitting the criteria for diagnosis are best treated with antidepressants.

336. Avoid suntan parlors.

337. Any white lesions in the mouth
should be checked by your doctor.

338. Pain in the ribs where they attach
to the breastbone is very common,
usually associated with tenderness
in that area, and successfully
treated with aspirin.

339. A tooth that has been completely
knocked out can be reimplanted.
Save the tooth in milk, call your
dentist, or get to the hospital.
Thirty minutes seems to be the
time limit.

340. Adolescent girls on a vegetarian diet need guidance from a registered dietitian. Most parents are not registered dietitians.

341. Make sure there's fluoride in your toothpaste if not in your drinking water.

342. You will handle stress better if you are physically fit.

343. Low-yield cigarettes are not safe. Quitting is the only way.

344. I have seen men laid up by bursitis
and men with widespread cancer of
the prostate put in 3,000 bales of
hay in a summer. Twenty years of
practice has taught me this:
Attitude is everything.

345. *Variability is the law of life, and as
no two faces are the same, so no two
bodies are alike, and no two
individuals react alike and behave
alike under the abnormal conditions
which we know as disease.*

Sir William Osler

346. About 20 percent of sexually active adolescents carry chlamydia infection. About 25 to 40 percent of sexually active adults in the United States show evidence of asymptomatic genital herpes infection. There are now good laboratory tests for both.

347. Transient loss of muscle function in an arm or a leg, or similar loss of sensation occurring suddenly and clearing completely within minutes to a few hours is always serious. It is called a *transient ischemic attack*, signals compromised circulation to a part of the brain, and warns of impending stroke. You must be seen for this.

348. To treat nosebleed: sit up, clamp your nose between your fingers for five minutes; if the bleeding then starts again, clamp continuously for ten minutes more; if you are unsuccessful, go to an emergency room.

349. The toll-free number for the Arthritis Foundation is: 1-800-283-7800.

350. The toll-free number for the American Parkinson Disease Association is: 1-800-223-2732.

351. Infection around the nail in its folds of skin can usually be cleared up with warm soaks. I like Epsom salts for this. If it is not improving within twenty-four hours, call your doctor.

352. Pleurisy is sudden chest pain with coughing or deep breathing. It can be a symptom of pneumonia or blood clot to the lung. Report this to your doctor.

353. Pneumonia usually produces a fever over 102°F—except in the elderly, when the temperature can be normal, and the patient very, very ill.

354. The cardinal symptom of "walking" pneumonia (in addition to fever, shortness of breath, and pleurisy) is a bothersome cough at night. Penicillin-type drugs are ineffective. Your doctor will treat you with tetracycline or erythromycin.

355. For topical medicines, ointments are superior to creams.

356. Teenage girls with appendicitis
lose their appetite, do not eat at all
during the day of the pain, usually
have a slight fever, and some
bowel irregularities. Teen girls
with mid-cycle ovulatory pain in
the right lower abdomen have none
of these symptoms.

357. Yes, you should reduce your fat consumption and eat more fruits, vegetables, and grains. But you knew this, didn't you?

358. Any canned food contained in a swollen can should be thrown away. Botulism can be fatal and is not destroyed by cooking.

359. If you are not pregnant, have controlled blood pressure, and have no problem with anxiety, insomnia, or heartburn, enjoy your coffee guilt-free. There are more important things to worry about.

360. Caffeine withdrawal can produce a headache from hell. Make sure that is not the cause of your headache before you panic and call the neurosurgeon.

361. Sports drinks and salt tablets are for the seven-figure athletes. Drink water, and bouillon if you feel you really need the salt replacement.

362. Merely buying expensive running shoes will not make you physically fit, any more than collecting books makes you learned.

363. In high school, way back when, the coaches fed us tea and toast before the game. That's still a great pregame meal. Fill up *after* you've won.

364. How in the world can you eat a
quarter of a pound of pecan pie and
gain three pounds??? Here's how:
You store the sugar as glycogen
and water, the pie crust as fat and
water. So you cheated. You're only
human. Keep at it. You'll get there.

365. Your doctor at hand is sometimes all the treatment you will need.

366. It's entirely normal to feel depressed for the first few weeks after delivery of a new baby. Don't feel guilty about it, for heaven's sake. It too will pass.

367. Psoriasis is that scaly, reddish rash you have noticed on others, most commonly affecting the knees, elbows, and scalp. It runs in families, only rarely affects the entire body, and is markedly improved by warm weather and sunlight.

368. Retinal detachment produces
blurred vision, flashes of light in
one eye, and floaters. Sometimes
visual images appear with wavy
lines. The detachment can be
repaired if caught early enough.
Consider these symptoms an
emergency.

369. Rheumatic fever results from untreated or inadequately treated strep infections. Thanks to antibiotics, it is a rare disease these days. But if you have a strep throat, take *all* of your antibiotics.

370. *As with eggs, there is no such thing as a poor doctor; doctors are either good or bad.*

Fuller Albright

371. Fungal infections of the toenails are not treated. The treatment is worse than the disease.

372. You are *not* getting old! Most male
impotence is caused by drugs and
medication. (And drugs include
excess alcohol . . .)

373. After serious illness, expect to be
depressed. It's a normal reaction.
It will pass. The End is not near.

374. *When the clever doctor fails, find one less clever.*

Proverb, Bechuanaland, South Africa

375. The best cure for the holiday
doldrums is a visit to a hospital on
Christmas Eve.

376. For arthritis of aging, try aspirin or
Tylenol® (acetaminophen) first. All
other "arthritis medicines" are
merely alternatives—neither
better nor worse.

377. *I watched what method Nature might take, with intention of subduing the symptom by treading in her footsteps.*
Thomas Sydenham, M.D. (1624–89)

378. When you are ready to quit smoking, use nicotine in gum or patches together with organized smoking cessation programs. Nothing else works as well.

379. Most things are better by morning.

380. Yes! By all means take these antioxidants. Each day:

- One gram of vitamin C
- 400 IU of vitamin E
- 25,000 IU of beta-carotene (vitamin A)

No more than that. No
multivitamins, no megavitamins,
no herbal extracts, no organic
formulations necessary. And no
additional vitamins or minerals
unless your doctor says so.

381. Confused about fats? Saturated, polyunsaturated, monounsaturated, butter, margarine, olive oil? Research is ongoing. All the answers are not yet in. Everyone's confused. But you can start with a blood test: a serum cholesterol. Then go from there.

382. Don't take iron supplements for anemia unless you are proven to have iron-deficiency anemia.

383. Most rashes are the result of an allergy. If generalized (all over the body), think medicines. Are you taking any pills you might now be allergic to? If localized (in one spot), think contact allergy from an external source. Common

culprits: fabric softeners, soaps
(all kinds), shampoos, cosmetics,
nickel (from those cheap earring
posts), deodorants, latex.

384. You can provoke a rash through allergy to one contact substance, then keep it going with something else. Example: a rash develops on your face. It's clear to you the makeup is to blame. You stop using it. The rash persists. So stop the

soaps, lotions, shampoos, creams,
etc. Just use hypoallergenic
(Basis®) soap. Rash still there?
Use an over-the-counter cortisone
cream (with a hypoallergenic base)
twice a day. Almost always, you'll
cure it. Money saved.

385. When do doctors worry about headaches? When a patient complains that it is new, un-relenting, localized at a point on the skull, or described as "the worst headache I have ever had." That's when. A story like that dictates a CAT scan or an MRI (types of sophisticated X-ray imaging).

386. Numbness and tingling in the hands and feet is *not* a symptom of multiple sclerosis. Multiple sclerosis produces a variety of neurological symptoms over time: weakness, double vision, imbalance, and vertigo in addition to abnormal sensation in one hand or one foot or one spot on the trunk or face.

387. Knee pain with locking, instability, and a feeling of a loose body requires outpatient surgery through a scope (arthroscopy). But for knee pain alone unresponsive to aspirin, see your primary doctor first. You may, by so doing, avoid unnecessary surgery.

388. When thinking about specialists, generalists, and high-tech medicine, remember this old saw: When all you have is a hammer, everything looks like a nail.

389. *Physicians are many in title but very few in reality.*

Hippocrates

390. Pain and swelling below the ear or under the tongue is from an infected salivary gland, usually obstructed by stone. You will need antibiotics and pain medication. The stone usually passes of its own accord.

391. Seasonal affective disorder is not a "yuppie" disease, but a genuine hormonally based depression occurring in the winter months. In Maine, we call it cabin fever. Physical activity, sunlight, and a winter vacation will help those who suffer from this recurring problem.

392. The Chinese pictogram for unhappiness depicts two women under one roof.

393. The most common cause of dry mouth is side effect from medication.

394. Diabetics: See an M.D. ophthalmologist every one to three years as a routine.

395. If your college-age child suddenly exhibits altruistic behavior through blood donation, he or she is probably seeking an HIV test.

396. Nothing dampens libido so effectively as children in the home.

397. Emergency treatment of shock hasn't changed since your scouting days: elevate the legs, warm the victim, put pressure on any bleeding, and call for help.

398. Treat sprains with RICE:
   *R*est, *I*ce, *C*ompression,
   *E*levation.

399. A sore tongue can be a symptom of
   food allergy.

400. Curvature of the spine is common in adolescent girls and easily spotted if looked for. Sharp school nurses frequently diagnose it. This is a condition better treated when caught early on.

401. Other than allergy, these can cause
a runny nose: cigarette smoke, air
pollutants, perfumes, nasal sprays,
some blood pressure medications,
birth-control pills, pregnancy,
aspirin, arthritis medication, and
sudden changes in ambient
temperature.

402. Oral contraceptives will not protect you against AIDS.

403. Most menstruating women require extra iron.

404. Occupational asthma can occur in bakers, dairy workers, dock workers, poultry handlers, laboratory technicians, pharmacists, food handlers, tobacco farmers, beauticians, carpenters, sawmill operators, brewers, nurses, printers, rug makers, dry cleaners, and snow crab workers. Among others.

405. The onset of bloody diarrhea after antibiotic use demands immediate medical attention.

406. Food intolerances—to lactose
sugar in milk, and to gluten
protein in breads —are not
uncommon. They can become
apparent in adulthood and can be
diagnosed with simple testing.
Symptoms are bowel cramping and
diarrhea associated with the foods.

407. To treat chronic constipation, add fiber, water, and exercise to your daily regimen.

408. A sty is that small abscess of an eyelash follicle. Apply hot soaks to it several times a day and it will usually drain on its own. *Never* squeeze it.

409. To treat a bad sunburn, soak in a cool tub to which some baking soda has been added. Then apply cold creams.

410. *Any fool can cut off a leg—it takes a surgeon to save one.*

George G. Ross

411. The first sign of syphilis is a *painless* red sore on the genitals, mouth, or rectum.

412. Increased redness and pus around a surgical wound is not normal procedure. These are signs of a wound infection and you need to be seen.

413. Amniocentesis can detect the
presence of Tay-Sachs disease in
the fetus. The disease is common
in French Canadians and
Ashkenazi Jews, very rare in
others.

414. Grinding your teeth at night (bruxism) is a sign of stress. Exercise, make love, read poetry, listen to music, and if necessary, wear a fitted dental guard at night to eliminate the problem.

415. Tennis elbow—pain and
tenderness on the bone at the
outside of the elbow—is common
in wood splitters, golfers,
carpenters, and . . . tennis players.
Don't just put up with it. Use a
forearm splint, then a forearm
strap, and do strengthening
exercises. A physical therapist can
advise.

416. Smoking, obesity, pregnancy, birth-control pills, estrogens, and long periods of inactivity make one prone to clots in the veins of the legs. This is a disease of truck drivers as well.

417. A whitish fungal infection of the mouth (with yeast organisms) can be the first overt sign of AIDS in an HIV-positive person.

418. Proscar® has *limited* application for enlargement of the prostate. Its heavy advertising is not warranted.

419. To treat early ingrown toenail, put
a piece of dental floss under the
nail corner.

420. Never use superabsorbent
tampons.

421. Peanut allergy is serious. You
never outgrow it. Peanut oil can be
found in the strangest of foods.
Always check. Always carry your
allergy kit with you.

422. If your best friend comes over for tea and:
- is depressed
- has evidence of multiple trauma in various stages of healing and,
- complains of vague aches and pains,

most likely she is a victim of domestic violence.

423. What are the signs of early Alzheimer's disease?

- impairment in the use of language, especially in writing and in the finding of words
- impaired recent memory, with remote memory preserved
- no changes in behavior, no tremor, no palsies, no urinary incontinence.

424. Thyroid cancer is curable. If you feel a lump in the front of your neck below your larynx, call your doctor.

425. Blacks are at greater risk for diabetes and hypertension. Get checked for these problems at least yearly.

426. Hypoglycemia the disease is extremely rare. If you tell your doctor you have symptoms from "low blood sugar" and she is skeptical, listen to her.

427. Women over forty require an annual breast examination and should perform monthly breast self-examination. At age fifty, add to this an annual mammography.

428. You can reduce flatus by reducing your milk intake.

429. If you are over fifty, have severe
aches and pains in the hips and
shoulders, have a scalp so tender it
hurts to brush your hair, have
headaches located in the temples,
have jaw pain severe enough to
prevent your chewing, have any or
all of these things, you have about

a 15 percent chance of going completely blind, irretrievably and forever. The condition is called *polymyalgia rheumatica.* It is easily diagnosed with a blood test, is easily treated successfully, and when so treated, blindness is always prevented.

430. When dining on a home-grown, home-fed pig, well-done is the only way to go.

431. Warts are caused by viruses. Scratching a wart spreads the virus, and the warts.

432. Long after Christmas has passed, a
doctor's office remembers the best
cookies.

433. The more estranged the family, the
more violently do its members
react to serious illness in the
family.

434. In an intensive care unit, the
doctor's best weapon against death
is a good nurse.

435. *Healing is a matter of time, but it is
sometimes also a matter of
opportunity.*

Hippocrates

436. Ringing in the ears can be a sign of: anemia, advancing age, under- or overactive thyroid, earwax, noise trauma, allergies, high blood pressure, or a side effect from medication, infection, or brain tumor.

437. The best initial treatment for foot
pain is not surgery, but rather the
best running shoes money can buy.
No matter what your age.

438. You will know an excellent physical examination when you have one.

439. Alcoholics as yet unwilling to abstain remain defensive.

440. The most dangerous drug on the college campus is alcohol.

441. With birches surrounding us for centuries, we have only now discovered that birch bark can treat melanoma. How are we doing with the rain forests?

442. Infertile women with obesity and hirsutism may have multiple cysts on the ovaries (Stein-Leventhal syndrome) and can have fertility restored with a simple surgical procedure.

443. If we want clean air and clean rivers for better health, we will have to pay more for paper. We can't have it both ways.

444. If you can't brush after a meal, chew sugarless gum to help clean your teeth.

445. Cleansing enemas are a relic from the past. They are not necessary for good health, and are not a home remedy for any disease.

446. Two reasons to get to the hospital
at once if you suspect a heart
attack:

- high risk of sudden death
- clot-dissolving drugs given
  early can limit the extent of the
  damage

447. Wait six months after a heart attack before undergoing elective surgery.

448. Almost all true stomach ulcers are caused by a bacterium (and not by stress, coffee, acid foods, or Mexican cuisine). There is a blood

test available to detect this
bacterium *(helicobacter pylori)*.
Antibiotics can eradicate this bug
and cure the ulcer. The incon-
venience of antacids and the
expense of "ulcer" medications
(e.g. Zantac®, or Tagamet®) are
unnecessary.

449. Rectal itching is very common. Its causes are many. First try hot bathes, hypoallergenic soap (Basis®), and avoidance of any other topical medications.

450. Let's say it again: Those "arthritis" medicines advertised so heavily—Motrin®, Advil®, Naprosyn®, Indocin®, Ansaid®, Nuprin®, Feldene®, Voltaren®, Anaprox®—have no advantage over aspirin, nor one over the other, and may cause serious side effects.

451. Impotence in women posthysterec-
tomy or postmenopause responds
well to estrogen therapy.

452. Hearing loss from noise is as
common as that from advancing
age. Loud, blaring, modern music
is a common cause.

453. The estimated prevalence of HIV infection among college students is about two students per thousand.

454. Treat acute diarrhea initially with Kaopectate®, then with Immodium®, then call your doctor. Bloody diarrhea is always serious.

455. The most common bleeding
tendency that runs in families is
called von Willebrand's Disease. It
is not serious, is not hemophilia, is
easily diagnosed, and its problems
are easily avoided. Not to worry.

456. Eat raw shellfish only in upscale restaurants. Otherwise, learn about hepatitis A.

457. Tattoo parlors are a source of hepatitis B.

458. Blood for transfusion is screened for hepatitis A and B, and for HIV infection.

459. If you carry genital herpes, you will not spread the disease if you do not have active ulcers or symptoms. Or if you use condoms.

460. The initial infection with HIV virus is marked by a flulike illness.

461. If you get near birds or bats in the Midwest and then experience cough and fever, get checked for a fungal disease called histoplasmosis.

462. Intense abdominal pain after a bout of drinking is not merely an upset stomach, but commonly an inflamed pancreas, and requires hospitalization.

463. If you are under treatment for high blood pressure and you develop chest pain, talk to your doctor immediately.

464. *Given one well-trained physician of the highest type he will do better work for a thousand people than ten specialists.*

William J. Mayo

465. If you have morning erections yet
are having difficulties performing
sexually, your impotence is
psychologically based.

466. If a loved one is terminally ill, try to get plenty of rest—use sleeping pills if necessary. The aftermath is far more arduous.

467. Severe eye pain with extreme
sensitivity to light has many
causes, all serious. See your
doctor immediately.

468. Dark-skinned people will sometimes get an overgrowth of scar tissue at an injury site. This is of cosmetic importance only and will not turn to cancer.

469. Legionnaires' disease spreads via heating and cooling systems. It is not contagious between people.

470. The large, soft, fatty tumors under the skin are called lipomas. They are harmless and never become cancerous.

471. Occasional acid reflux or heartburn is not a serious problem.

472. Never take someone else's medication. Never.

473. To prevent *osteoporosis* (thinning of the bones with hip fractures, dowager's hump), stop smoking, get regular, weight-bearing exercise, take hormonal replacement therapy during and after menopause, be moderate with alcohol, and take four to six flavored Tums® per day.

474. Infection of the skin itself, cellulitis, produces a sudden redness and swelling of the skin, usually over the leg below the knee. The redness spreads rapidly and there is usually fever and swollen glands in the groin. Antibiotics that day! Don't delay.

475. Most neck and shoulder pain is from wear and tear on the bones in the neck and is not serious. Treat with a soft collar, hot showers, better posture, and massage therapy if you can get it.

476. A corneal abrasion from trauma or from ill-fitting contact lenses produces intense pain, aversion to bright light, copious tearing of the eye, blurred vision, spasm of the eyelid, and a red eye. Get it seen immediately.

477. Pain in the chest where the ribs attach to the breastbone is called costochondritis. The pain is sharp, and there is pronounced tenderness in the area. The pain worsens with movement and with breathing, and is easily treated with aspirin or ibuprofen. The condition is not serious and completely resolves.

478. For minor dandruff, and "dandruff
of the chest" (seborrheic
dermatitis), use Selsun®. Lather
up, leave it on overnight, and rinse
it off the next morning. Do this
twice a week only, until the
problem is controlled.

479. Vaginal pain and discomfort after menopause, with pain on intercourse, can be treated with topical estrogen creams.

480. Pregnancy developing outside the uterus is always serious. The early signs are: a positive pregnancy test followed by a heavy painful period or vaginal bleeding or spotting, and lower abdominal cramping and pain. An abdominal echo (ultrasound) can make the diagnosis.

481. A painful, enlarged, tender testis, with fever and a tender scrotum means infection of the structures adjacent to the testis. Antibiotic therapy is mandatory. Call your doctor.

482. For generalized dry skin, try Alpha-Keri Bath Oil® applied directly from the bottle.

483. Skin-So-Soft® will repel mosquitoes and black flies (gnats) for about twenty minutes. Then they resume feeding.

484. Lumpy breasts, especially tender and painful just before menses, with lumps that enlarge at that time, comprise fibrocystic breast disease. It does not predispose to cancer. Effective therapy includes ibuprofen, vitamin B-6, vitamin E, and yes, kelp tablets (containing iodine).

485. Some women *do* ache all over. Pain and tenderness in the muscles and tendons of the hips, low back, neck, shoulders, chest, and thighs (but not the joints), together with fatigue and stiffness is called fibromyalgia and is not a psychiatric illness. Treat with aspirin or ibuprofen, a daily exercise program, and weight loss if necessary.

486. If you are prone to pustules and boils on the skin, bathe with an antibacterial soap, such as Clearasil® or Betadyne®.

487. B-12 shots are a placebo and a waste of money unless you have proven pernicious anemia.

488. A whitened digit occurring with brief cold exposure is neither frostbite nor gangrene. Called Raynaud's sign, it may be innocent, or a marker of other disease. Talk to your doctor.

489. Swollen gums that bleed easily, coupled with bad breath, are from gingivitis. You need a dental appointment and antibiotics.

490. Chronic glaucoma is absolutely painless. And leads to blindness. The only way to beat it is with an eye checkup.

491. Heart palpitations from stress, caffeine, and nicotine are almost always benign in an otherwise healthy heart. But get this checked if you eliminate the apparent cause and they persist.

492. If you are prone to spells of rapid heartbeat, you can abort them quickly by plunging your face in a sink full of cold water. It's called the diving reflex.

493. Avoid heatstroke by drinking water *before* you are thirsty.

494. Cramping pain in the right upper
abdomen, often going through to
the back, tenderness in that area,
nausea and vomiting, and possibly
a slight fever—these signal a gall
bladder attack.

495. Do not assume that all dementia is Alzheimer's—and beware of such a casual diagnosis. Treatable dementias can come from B-12 deficiency, infection, benign brain tumor, clot on the brain as a consequence of a (very minor) fall, endocrine (glandular) disorders, depression, schizophrenia, and high spinal fluid pressure.

496. Cirrhosis—scarring of the liver—can be caused by as little as six ounces of alcohol a day when consumed steadily over several years.

497. Corns are treated easily. Remove
the source of pressure. (Change
shoes!) Apply nonprescription 10
percent salicylic ointment and
cover. Repeat until gone.

498. The three cardinal symptoms of diabetes are increased thirst, increased appetite, and increased urination.

499. Pregnancy after age forty-five carries a one in twenty risk of Down's syndrome in the baby. Diagnosis can be made through analysis of amniotic fluid during the pregnancy.

500. Take this book to your next
doctor's appointment if you wish.
You will not upset a good doctor by
so doing.

Dr. LaCombe practiced general internal medicine for twenty years in rural Maine, is Director Emeritus of the **American Board of Internal Medicine,** a Regent of the **American College of Physicians,** and associate editor of the **Annals of Internal Medicine** and the **American Journal of Medicine.**

Bibliography/Research Material for
THE POCKET DOCTOR

American Journal of Medicine, vols. 98–99, 1995.

Annals of Internal Medicine, vols. 120–23, 1994–95

Cecil-Loeb Textbook of Internal Medicine, 19th ed., W.B. Saunders, 1992.

Harrison's Principles of Internal Medicine, 13th ed., McGraw-Hill, 1994.

Harvard Health Letter, vols. 19–20, 1994–95.

Journal of the American Medical Association, vols. 273–74, 1995.

Lancet, vols. 343–46, 1994–95.

New England Journal of Medicine, vols. 330–33, 1994–95.

Principles of Ambulatory Medicine, 2nd ed., Williams & Wilkins, N.Y., 1986.

Scientific American Medicine, 1978–95, Scientific American Inc.

INDEX

INDEX

INDEX

INDEX

INDEX

INDEX

INDEX

INDEX

INDEX

INDEX